Maria Socorro Cardoso dos Santos
Gizelda M. Silva
Jaques Waisberg

Elderly health

Maria Socorro Cardoso dos Santos
Gizelda M. Silva
Jaques Waisberg

Elderly health

Physical and mental activity to help treat depression in the elderly

ScienciaScripts

Imprint

Any brand names and product names mentioned in this book are subject to trademark, brand or patent protection and are trademarks or registered trademarks of their respective holders. The use of brand names, product names, common names, trade names, product descriptions etc. even without a particular marking in this work is in no way to be construed to mean that such names may be regarded as unrestricted in respect of trademark and brand protection legislation and could thus be used by anyone.

Cover image: www.ingimage.com

This book is a translation from the original published under ISBN 978-613-9-65443-7.

Publisher:
Sciencia Scripts
is a trademark of
Dodo Books Indian Ocean Ltd. and OmniScriptum S.R.L publishing group

120 High Road, East Finchley, London, N2 9ED, United Kingdom
Str. Armeneasca 28/1, office 1, Chisinau MD-2012, Republic of Moldova, Europe
Printed at: see last page
ISBN: 978-620-7-77751-8

SUMMARY

SUMMARY

In Brazil and around the world, ageing is a reality. It is now known that this is due to changes related to the fall in fertility and the ageing of the population. This leads to demographic and epidemiological changes that alter the population's health profile. The emergence of chronic degenerative diseases has led to changes in the morbidity profile of the elderly. Depression is one of these chronic conditions and is associated with functional limitations, compromising the well-being of the elderly. It is a morbidity that is difficult to measure and its causes vary from psychosocial to genetic and biological factors. This is an exploratory, interpretative, qualitative study based on field research and using content analysis. In addition to identifying the incidence and prevalence of depression among the elderly, we opted for a qualitative study to identify whether those who have or have had depression accepted practicing physical and mental activity as an aid to treating depression. We also sought to answer specific questions that cannot be quantified. The proposal was to promote reflection on depression in the elderly, with the aim of identifying the functional impact of depression on them, characterizing the profile of elderly people attending a Basic Health Unit located in the southern region of the municipality of Sao Paulo, and identifying those who had depression. We also analyzed the impact of social relationships and physical activities on the elderly as factors that promote improvements in depression and propose physical and mental activity as an aid in its treatment. To carry out the study, we randomly invited 50 elderly people aged 60 or over who had or had not suffered from depression. Based on the data collected by applying a questionnaire made up of objective and open-ended questions, we found concrete evidence that elderly people who practiced some kind of physical activity had a lower prevalence of depression. In this way, we believe that physical and mental activity is very important both in prevention and after the onset of depression, positively influencing coping with depression. We also found that the majority of elderly people who had suffered from depression showed a significant improvement once they started taking part in physical and mental activity. This proves that physical activity leads directly to mental exercise, thus helping to treat depression in the elderly.

Keywords: Depression; Physical activity; Elderly.

1   INTRODUCTION AND JUSTIFICATION

According to the World Health Organization (WHO), since the 1990s, depression has occupied a prominent position on the list of public health problems, and is currently considered to be the fourth most expensive of all diseases worldwide for government coffers. In 2010, depression was second only to ischemic heart disease (WHO, 2006).

By 2020, depression will be the second most common disease in developed countries and the first in developing countries (NASCIMENTO, 1999; LAFER & AMARAL, 2000).

According to Angst (1999 cited in Comer, 2003), depression is a very common illness characterized by long-lasting episodes, high chronicity, relapses and recurrences, psychosocial and physical damage and a high risk of suicide, not to mention deaths caused by complications and associated risk factors.

Currently, there are an average of two million new depressed people a year in the world. Recent studies show that in Brazil alone, more than 10 million people are suffering from this illness, so depression is considered to be one of the greatest threats to the balance of well-being in the new millennium (WHO, 2006).

For Camon (2001), depression emerges as the result of a global inhibition of the person which significantly affects the function of the mind, alters the way the person sees the world, feels reality, understands things and expresses their emotions.

In this way, depression is considered to be a disease of the body as a whole, which affects the human being as a whole, without separating the psychic, social and physical.

Still according to this author, despair about life, anguish, the desire for an end, death as a constant presence, fear as an ally of existence, abandonment of self-esteem, suicide as a proposal, among other signs, express the pain of the depressed individual.

Sougey, Azevedo and Taveira (2001) believe that when suffering from depression, the individual is faced with feelings and thoughts of pessimism, helplessness, deep sadness, apathy, lack of initiative, physical discontent, difficulty in organizing and flowing ideas, impaired cognitive judgment, among other symptoms.

Studies on depression reveal a large number of illnesses in general terms, especially those referred to as mental illness, which is distorted from its real meaning. In common sense, it refers to everything from psychological alterations and serious psychiatric disorders to mood or character fluctuations (COUTINHO, 2001).

For Stoppe and Segal (1998), there are currently three different uses of the term "depression":

- For lay people, they describe depression as an unexplained sadness and discouragement, but they are not aware that this event is necessarily related to a disorder or illness;

- For psychiatry, referring to a symptom usually related to depressed mood; and the use to define a syndrome, based on a set of symptoms;

- Some studies have reported that people who experience conflict, loss, lack of affection, physical limitations, family problems and other adversities in their daily lives are more susceptible to suffering from this syndrome.

It should be noted, however, that not all individuals, even if they share similar lifestyles and situations, develop depressive symptoms. So how do they differ? Specific literature points to the existence of factors that make some people more predisposed than others, including susceptibility, gender, heredity, age and the influence of the environment (CANON, 2001; LAFER and AMARAL, 2000).

In relation to age, which is the subject of this paper, the "elderly" go through a natural process of vulnerability that is relevant to their personal and social trajectory.

This process most often stems from factors that can trigger depression. The factors can be referred to as biological, psychological and social, experienced over the course of the elderly person's life, associated with loss, family breakdown, loneliness or even their way of life, and can detect signs of depression in the face of frailty in the elderly, characterizing the etiological factors of the disease (WAGNER, 2015).

The research topic was chosen as a result of my academic training as a nurse, during which the stages presented here were experienced.

The first stage took place in a theoretical context, where I was able to get involved with scientific themes by means of data in accordance with the norms evidenced by theoretical references supported by reliable databases, as well as by taking part in congresses, lectures and multi- and interdisciplinary discussions.

The second stage was related between training and professional practice, which was established between the theoretical context learned in the classroom, during the undergraduate nursing course between 2002 and 2006, where depression was already discussed and pointed out as one of the major public health problems in the face of the social transformations that have occurred in recent decades, together with the professional experience acquired as a professional working in the health area.

In a final, third stage, acquired in the personal sphere, in the family context, there were situations of confrontation with sadness, loss, anguish, where amidst an internal restlessness an interest in the capacity for resilience in the face of depression was awakened and with unknowns to identify the competence of being a nurse in this context.

I would like to emphasize the importance of the gerontology subject in the training of nurses, as well as the day-to-day work placement where students can assess and promote care for people at risk or in a situation of depression in order to restore their mental health.

Thus, I seek to understand depression in the elderly, and whether physical activity can be promoted as a care proposal to promote treatment and self-care for depression, based on evidence.

2 OBJECTIVES

2.1 General Objective

To identify the functional impact of depression on elderly people attending a Basic Health Unit located in the southern region of the State of Sao Paulo.

2.2 Specific Objectives

a) To characterize the profile of the elderly attending a Basic Health Unit - UBS located in the southern region of the municipality of Sao Paulo, identifying those with depression;

b) To identify the adherence of elderly people with depression to the practice of physical activity as an aid to their treatment;

c) Analyzing the impact of social relationships and physical activities on the elderly as complementary factors in improving depression.

3 CONTEXTUALIZING THE TOPIC

The aging of the Brazilian population is related to a worldwide phenomenon. According to the United Nations (UN), in 2013, its latest technical report entitled "World Population Forecasts", prepared by the Department of Economic and Social Affairs, states that in the next 43 years the number of people over 60 will be three times greater than it is today. The elderly will account for a quarter of the projected world population, or around 2 billion individuals (out of a total of 9.2 billion). According to the criteria of the World Health Organization (WHO), elderly people in developing countries are those aged 60 and over and those aged 65 and over in developed countries.

In 1998, life expectancy in developed countries was 70.6 years for men and 78.4 for women, rising to 87.5 and 92.5 years respectively by 2050.

In developing countries, it will be 82 years for men and 86 for women, 21 years more than the current 62.1 and 65.2. This phenomenon is due to the reduction in fertility and mortality rates (BERQUÓ, 2006).

For the same author, this condition leads to demographic and epidemiological changes that alter the health profile of the population, where the emergence of chronic-degenerative diseases causes changes in the morbidity profile of the elderly.

Depression is one of these chronic conditions and is associated with functional limitations, compromising the well-being of the elderly. It is a morbidity that is difficult to measure and its causes vary from psychosocial, genetic to biological factors.

3.1 Depression

According to Kaplan et al. (1997), in the general population, depression has a prevalence of around 15%. In elderly people living in the community, Edwards (2003) pointed out that this prevalence is between 2 and 14% and, according to Pamerlee et al. (1989), in elderly people living in long-term care facilities, it is as high as 30%.

In the elderly, depression has been characterized as a syndrome involving numerous clinical, etiopathogenic and treatment aspects. When it starts late, it is often associated with general medical illnesses and structural and functional brain abnormalities. If left untreated, depression increases the risk of clinical morbidity and mortality, especially in elderly people hospitalized with general illnesses (PAMERLEE, 1989).

The causes of depression in the elderly form part of a broad set of components involving genetic factors, life events such as bereavement and abandonment, and incapacitating illnesses, among others. It should be emphasized that depression in the elderly often arises in a context of loss of quality of life associated with social isolation and the onset of serious clinical illnesses. Chronic and disabling illnesses are risk factors for depression. Feelings of frustration at the unfulfilled aspirations of life and the subject's own history marked by progressive losses such as the loss of a partner, emotional ties and the ability to work, as well as abandonment, social isolation, the inability to re-engage in productive activity, the lack of social return on educational investment, retirement that undermines the minimum resources for survival, are factors that compromise quality of life and predispose the elderly to the development of depression (PACHECO, 2002).

3.2 Neurobiological Aspects of Depression

Identifying the onset of depression and the specific conditions in which it occurs is extremely important for the etiological diagnosis of depression and its co-morbidities, as well as for treatment and prognosis. Thus, elderly patients whose depression began early in life and continues into old age tend to have a significant genetic component. On the other hand, in those whose depression started after the age of 65, genetic interference tends to be less intense and neurobiological phenomena tend to be more important. Obviously, the action of psychic components that accumulate throughout life cannot be excluded (FREITAS and ROCHA, 2006).

Certain neurobiological factors can lead to late-onset depression by increasing the risk and vulnerability of the elderly to depression, such as neuroendocrine alterations (reduced response to thyroid stimulating hormone), neurotransmitter alterations (reduced serotonergic and noradrenergic activity), vascular alterations and processes of degeneration of cortical and subcortical circuits responsible for processing and elaborating affective and emotional life. The decreased production of serotonin by the raphe nuclei and the decrease in receptors for these neurotransmitters represent factors of vulnerability to depression in the elderly (FREITAS and ROCHA 2006).

Impairment of the basal ganglia, particularly the caudate nucleus and thalamus, has been associated with late-onset depression (GREENWALD et al., 1996; 1998).

Hypofrontality, verified by functional neuroimaging, such as brain SPECT (Single Photon Emission Computerized Tomography), showing a reduction in prefrontal cortical activity, has also been correlated with late-onset depression. In depression with psychotic symptoms (delusions and hallucinations), structural and functional neuroimaging resources can be applied. Kim et al. (1999) carried out a comparative study of the volumetry of various brain structures, using magnetic resonance imaging, between two groups -   19 elderly people with depression accompanied by symptoms

and 26 elderly people with depression but no psychotic symptoms. The researchers found significantly smaller volumes in the prefrontal cortical regions in the group of depressed patients with delusions. In the elderly, depression with psychotic symptoms, anxiety, irritability and emotional instability tend to predict the onset of behavioral disorders, especially aggression and psychomotor agitation.

Depression in the elderly usually manifests itself through frequent physical complaints associated with general medical illnesses, especially those which cause prolonged suffering, leading to physical dependence and loss of autonomy, and which induce hospitalization or institutionalization (FREITAS, 2006).

. The same author states that depression in these patients aggravates general medical illnesses and increases mortality. Despite its high prevalence in general medical illnesses, depression has not been properly diagnosed and treated.

Often, depressive symptoms are confused with general medical illness itself or as a "normal" consequence of ageing, and are not given much consideration. Depression and general medical illness have a reciprocal influence on the patient's clinical development. In some specific conditions, frequent in the elderly.

The main diseases that lead to depression in the elderly include Parkinson's disease (40 to 60%), Alzheimer's disease (30 to 40%), stroke (30 to 60%), Huntington's disease (30 to 40%), multiple sclerosis (20 to 60%) and epilepsy (10 to 50%). Conditions such as Cushing's syndrome, hypothyroidism, diabetes mellitus, heart disease and autoimmune diseases also have a high prevalence of depression (COLE and BELLAVANE, 1997; EVANS et al., 1997; PRINCE et al., 1998). It should be remembered that centrally acting drugs can cause depressive symptoms, such as anti-hypertensive drugs (alpha-methyldopa, clonidine, nifedipine, propranolol, digoxin), antiparkinsonian drugs (L-dopa, amantadine), benzodiazepines (diazepam and others), as well as corticoids (FREITAS and ROCHA 2006).

It should also be noted that prolonged periods of pain, compromised nutrition, weight loss and factors arising from physical illnesses that lead to reduced autonomy and loss of physical mobility contribute decisively to the onset of depression. Patients in these conditions tend to develop psychotic symptoms characterized by delusions of nullity and that their body is dying. Fear of the progression of the physical illness, the loss of dignity and the fear of becoming a burden to family members are also psychological phenomena that accompany the impairment of physical condition (FREITAS and ROCHA, 2006).

The depressed patient decreases self-care, refuses to eat or follow the doctor's recommendations, and remains confined to bed for longer or has little physical mobility. These factors, combined with general clinical weakness, can reduce immunity, making them more vulnerable to infectious processes (FREITAS and ROCHA, 2006).

The disease also affects cognitive functions, leading to the appearance of depressive disorders, which is considered a risk factor for the subsequent development of dementia. Some studies suggest that 50% of patients with depression develop dementia within five years (FREITAS and ROCHA, 2006).

The comorbidity of depression and dementia contributes to the impairment of their functional capacities. Depression can lead to temporary alterations in cognitive functions, often making it difficult to make a differential diagnosis between this condition and dementia. On the other hand, in many patients, the onset of Alzheimer's-type dementia is accompanied by depressive symptoms. In addition, there is an association between depressive symptoms and impaired cognitive functions in the elderly, with or without dementia. Memory complaints are common in depressed patients, traditionally suggesting the emergence of the term "depressive pseudodementia". According to Stoppe Jr and Louza Neto (1999), the reciprocal relationship between depression and dementia manifests itself as follows:

a) Depression in dementia: depressive symptoms are an integral part of the dementia process;

b) Dementia with depression: coexistence of both phenomena, with depressive symptoms occurring in the context of pre-existing dementia;

c) Depression with cognitive impairment: depression evolves with cognitive difficulties, particularly concentration and recent memory;

d) Dementia in depression: where cognitive impairment results from the depressive process ("depressive pseudodementia").

According to Angelotti (2001), the aim of treating depression in the elderly is to reduce the psychological suffering caused by this illness, reduce the risk of suicide, improve the patient's general condition and ensure a better quality of life.

According to the same author, the treatment not only of depression, but of other neuropsychiatric illnesses in the elderly, is a challenge that involves specialized intervention such as psychotherapy, psychopharmacological intervention and, when necessary, electroconvulsive therapy.

The author also mentions that the therapeutic role of physical activity should be analyzed in a specific section, where initially there is a need to identify factors that could be triggering the onset of a depressive process, or even aggravating existing depression. It is therefore pertinent to check whether the patient has any clinical illnesses that are related to depression and to see if the use of any medication (anti-inflammatory, antihypertensive, insomnia medication, etc.) is not leading to the onset of depressive symptoms. Next, psychological and psychosocial aspects should be investigated, such as bereavement, social isolation, abandonment and other factors that tend to trigger depressive symptoms. The study draws attention to the fact that psychotherapeutic intervention should preferably be carried out by professionals who specialize in the elderly. This helps to identify the factors that trigger the depressive process, contributing to guidance for family members, carers and the patient themselves. Activities such as occupational therapy, participation in artistic and leisure activities also play a role in the treatment of depressed elderly people (ANGELOTTI, 2001).

According to Angelotti (2001), the psychotherapeutic intervention that is particularly suitable for the elderly is called brief psychotherapy, because this modality, as well as minimizing the patient's psychological suffering, helps depressed elderly people to reorganize their life plans. It is a prospective therapy, focused on the present and the future, usually lasting six months. When the symptoms of depression put the patient's clinical condition at risk and when psychic suffering is significant, psychopharmacological intervention is necessary. Second-generation antidepressants are recommended, as they are safer drugs for the elderly.

Thus, the author states that untreated depression puts the patient's life at risk and greatly increases their suffering, as seen above, and there is no justification for not treating depression.

According to Freitas and Rocha (2006), the psychopharmacological treatment of depression in the elderly depends essentially on the patient's tolerability profile in relation to antidepressants. Selective serotonin reuptake inhibitors (SSRIs) are the first choice, especially citalopram and sertraline. Of the drugs in this category, these two have been the most studied in the elderly population. Paroxetine and fluoxetine, as well as others less common in the elderly, such as venlafaxine, have also been prescribed. In general, tricyclic antidepressants are not the first choice for elderly patients due to adverse effects, mainly anticholinergic. When it is necessary to prescribe a drug of this class, nortriptyline is recommended, starting with low doses and increasing them cautiously.

These authors emphasized that attention should be paid to the adverse effects of prescription drugs and the risk of drug interactions. Due to the presence of various illnesses that commonly affect the elderly, they tend to use several drugs, with a high risk of drug interactions and potentiation of adverse effects. In particular, drugs that produce or potentiate anticholinergic effects, postural hypotension, disturbances in the cardiac conduction system and delirium should be avoided. Combining psychopharmacological treatment with psychotherapy has shown good results. When the patient is at imminent risk of suicide and a rapid response is required, in catatonic conditions that do not respond to drug treatment and when the patient cannot tolerate psychopharmaceuticals, electroconvulsive therapy (ECT) is a valuable and safe option for the treatment of depression. Occasionally, there may be episodes of delirium and cognitive disorders, which are generally transient. It should be noted that electroconvulsive therapy can only be carried out within the parameters set by the Federal Council of Medicine, including ECT in a hospital environment, under general anesthesia and with a specialized team, respecting the patient's general clinical condition. Absolute contraindications to ECT are intracranial hypertension and the occurrence of acute myocardial infarction (3 months) or stroke (6 months). Obviously, a complete clinical examination of the patient and laboratory tests are recommended before the procedure is carried out, in order to check for other contraindications (DAS GUPTA, 2001).

3.3 Senescence and senility

Senescence refers to "old age" itself, in which there is a slow and gradual physical and mental decline, initially quite moderate, i.e. senescence is natural ageing (FREITAS and ROCHA, 2006).

Senility is characterized by faster physical decline accompanied by mental disorganization with altered cognitive functioning and memory loss, i.e. it is a pathological disorder associated with old age, but it does not mean old age itself. Therefore, senility corresponds to the psychopathological aspects of old age, which do not necessarily manifest themselves in the last phase of life (FREITAS ROCHA, 2006).

3.4 Theories of Ageing

Efforts have been made in various areas of human knowledge to understand the ageing process, especially anthropology, psychology and sociology. Theories of ageing began to be systematized in the 1960s, making up the first generation, and proposed universal application models. The theories of disengagement and activity are part of this initial process, making up the sociological theories of ageing. Because of their importance, they are all used, even if they are partial. The unit of analysis in this generation of theories is the individual, focusing on social roles and norms of adjustment to ageing (PY and TREIN, 2002).

We also have the theory of modernization. In order to better understand the importance of these theories in the ageing process, we will talk specifically about these three theories.

> **Disengagement theory** - this theory tries to explain the ageing process by understanding that older people who have tried to remain active have suffered an intimate conflict, because the desire to expand their living space is contradictory to the end of life. He understands that the elderly would like certain forms of isolation, the reduction of social contacts (disconnection), and that by doing so they would feel happy and satisfied, with greater well-being. This disconnection or disengagement would happen of the individual's own free will and would be an inevitable process. This

disengagement would also occur through society, which would free the elderly person from their social roles and obligations. A positive aspect of the theory is that the elderly person, on disengaging, would have a period of greater freedom, not having to abide by certain social norms (LEHR, 1980).

> **Activity theory** - This theory still influences the social movements of the elderly and guides projects in the area of leisure and non-formal education. These projects use as their central proposition the assumption that "social activity is in and of itself beneficial and produces greater satisfaction with life" (SIQUEIRA, 2002). In other words, physical and mental activity is the means by which the elderly achieve a better quality of life. It would therefore be interesting to maintain the activity levels of the earlier stages of life, as this would lead to successful ageing. Happiness and satisfaction in old age would go hand in hand (SIQUEIRA , 2002).

> **Modernization theory** - Modernization theory was presented by Cowgill and Holmes in 1972 and revised by Cowgill in 1974, describing the relationship between modernization and changes in the social roles and status of older people. The concept of modernization is associated with the process of industrialization, which leads to structural changes in societies, in a particular way, considering the historical and cultural context. The main argument is that the status of the elderly is directly related to the level of industrialization of society.

The central argument of these theories strengthens the idea that the status of the elderly is directly linked to the degree of industrialization of society. It defines the decline in status as the reduction in leadership roles, power and influence, as well as the withdrawal of the elderly from life and their community. In a way, this theory signals a concern about the exclusion of the elderly.

3.5 Levels of Ageing

It can be said that human ageing occurs on three different levels: biological, psychological and social.

Biological ageing involves physiological, anatomical, biochemical and hormonal changes, accompanied by a gradual decline in the body's capacities (FREITAS and ROCHA 2006).

Psychological ageing is expressed in people's behaviors (overt and covert) towards themselves or others, linked to changes in attitude and limitations in general capacities. These behaviors result in the occurrence of maladaptations, readaptations and readjustments of behavioral repertoires in the face of life's demands (FREITAS and ROCHA, 2006).

For the above authors, social ageing is related to the social norms or events that control, according to an age criterion, the performance of certain activities or tasks by the age group, and which give meaning to each person's life. As an example, we can mention: marriage is an event that usually takes place in the years of youth or early adulthood. The birth of children is more common between the ages of eighteen and thirty.

Making ageing a healthy stage of life is a major challenge for all areas of knowledge, including adding physical and mental activity to the daily lives of the elderly, and consequently giving quality of life to this population, which not only has the chance to live longer, but deserves to live with quality, dignity and above all, stimulating self-esteem to overcome small challenges (SANTARÉM, 2002).

3.6 The Relationship of Depression to the Elderly Patient

Some studies have shown that the clinical recognition of depression in the elderly was a milestone in the late 1960s and early 1970s, which in turn has also been controversial in terms of its diagnosis, making it difficult to recognize at this vital stage of human ageing (PAPALÉO NETTO, 1996).

The author points out that despite its recognized existence, depression in the elderly remains a major challenge for researchers who deal with this problem.

According to Valla and Bergeron (1993), the clinical recognition of this syndrome in the elderly is quite complex.

On the one hand, the symptoms are often attributed to genetic, social, degenerative brain processes and physical illnesses that contribute in varying proportions. On the other hand, older people are more susceptible to depression, especially when they lose their self-esteem and begin to see themselves as worthless, a burden on society and their families.

Living with loneliness, loss of meaning in life, renunciation and giving up are constant challenges in the ageing process. From an epidemiological point of view, it is estimated that around 15% of the elderly have some symptoms of depression, 2% of which are severe (LOUZÂ, NETO, 2000).

In some populations (hospitalized or institutionalized) the frequency is higher, reaching 5% to 13% of hospitalized patients and 12% to 16% of nursing home residents (DAS GUPA, 2001).

The incidence of depression is higher in nursing home populations or in acute hospitals than in the community (CALDAS and COLS,1994).

The rates of depressive symptoms in these populations are 31% and 23% respectively. Around 10% of elderly people in nursing homes develop a depressive episode within a year. What is known is that various situations can lead to depression, and that preventive diagnosis is necessary, mainly to avoid an acute onset.

According to BALLONE (2001), once diagnosed, treatment should be based on biological and psychosocial aspects. With the significant progress of research into the phenomenon of depression, various theoretical approaches have been researched and analyzed, some focusing more on the organic aspects, others on the psychological aspects.

However, this author adds that because of its complexity, and because it is prolix and multifaceted, to explain it from a particular viewpoint is to establish, at the very least, reductionist concepts that fail to take into account the plurality and complexity of the phenomenon.

3.7 Epidemiological Data on Depression in the Elderly in Brazil and Worldwide

Population ageing is one of the most notorious phenomena in the world today, bringing with it cultural, social and political repercussions. Brazil is a rapidly ageing country. Life expectancy increased from 33 to 68 years during the 20th century. According to the latest National Household Sample Survey (PNAD 2012), the elderly population exceeds 17 million, corresponding to approximately 10% of the Brazilian population. Projections for 2020 estimate 32 million, placing Brazil sixth in the world in terms of the number of elderly people. The progressive increase in life expectancy implies an increase in morbidity due to chronic non-communicable diseases, which are often disabling and which account for the majority of health expenditure in developed countries. Elderly depression, for example, is a major public health problem due to its high prevalence, frequent association with chronic diseases, negative impact on quality of life and risk of suicide. Approximately 15% to 20% of non-institutionalized elderly people have depressive symptoms. Comorbidity between physical and mental illnesses is of great interest, and it is generally accepted that the presence of an organic pathology increases the risk of psychiatric disorders (BRASIL, 2012).

Research has shown that clinical illnesses can contribute to the pathogenesis of depression through direct effects on brain function or through psychological or psychosocial effects. This association can be seen in a bidirectional way: depression precipitating chronic illnesses and chronic illnesses exacerbating depressive symptoms. This complex relationship has important implications for both the management of chronic illnesses and the treatment of depression.

3.8 Clinical aspects of depression and diagnosis

The diagnosis of depression goes through several stages: a detailed anamnesis with the patient and family members or caregivers, a thorough psychiatric examination, a general clinical examination, a neurological assessment, identification of adverse effects of medication, laboratory tests and neuroimaging. These are valuable procedures for diagnosing depression, psychopharmacological intervention and prognosis, especially given the higher prevalence of comorbidities and the greater risk of death. In elderly patients, in addition to the common symptoms, depression is usually accompanied by somatic complaints, hypochondria, low self-esteem, feelings of worthlessness, dysphoric mood, self-deprecating tendencies, altered sleep and appetite, paranoid ideation and recurrent thoughts of suicide. It should be remembered that in depressed patients the risk of suicide is twice as high as in non-depressed patients (PEARSON and BROWN, 2000). The symptoms (Table 1) are generally associated with the presence of physical illnesses or the use of medication.

Table 1. Symptoms of depression in the elderly

Mood symptoms	Neurovegetative symptoms	Symptoms Cognitive	Psychotic symptoms
Depressed/dysphoric Irritability Sadness Discouragement Feeling abandoned Feeling worthless Decreased self-esteem Social withdrawal/solidation Anhedonia and disinterest Self-deprecating ideas Ideas of death Suicide attempts	Inappetence Weight loss Sleep disturbance Loss of energy Psychomotor slowdown Psychomotor restlessness Hypochondria Unspecific pains	Difficulty -concentration memory - slow thinking	-Paranoid ideas -Delusions of ruin Delusions of death Commanding hallucinations of suicide

Source: Adapted from: Benjamin James Sadock, 2003.

3.9 Public Policies on Healthy Ageing

It is a fact that, with the increase in population ageing, it has also become one of the greatest challenges facing contemporary public health, with the search for the development and implementation of new public health policies, as well as the use of existing ones so that they can meet the needs of this new population (BRASIL, 2007).

The phenomenon of ageing first occurred in developed countries, but recently it has been in developing countries that the ageing of the population has been most pronounced. In Brazil, the number of elderly people (60 years old) rose from 3 million in 1960, to 7 million in 1975 and 14 million in 2002 (an increase of 500% in forty years) and it is estimated that it will reach 32 million in 2020 (BRASIL, 2007).

In countries like Belgium, for example, it took a hundred years for the elderly population to double in size and with this increase in the volume of the elderly population, the population pyramid showed the emergence of diseases typical of ageing, which are gaining greater expression in society as a whole. One of the results of this dynamic is a growing demand for health services. This is one of the current challenges (BRASIL, 2007).

The elderly consume more health services, hospital admissions are more frequent and bed occupancy times are longer when compared to other age groups. In general, the illnesses of the elderly are chronic and multiple, lasting several years and requiring constant monitoring, permanent care, continuous medication and increasingly complex periodic examinations (BRASIL, 2007).

Undoubtedly, one of humanity's greatest achievements has been the increase in life expectancy, which has been accompanied by a substantial improvement in the health parameters of populations, although these achievements are far from being distributed equally in different countries and socio-economic contexts (BRASIL, 2007).

What was once the privilege of a few, reaching old age, is now normal even in the poorest countries. This major achievement of the 20th century is, however, becoming a major challenge for the new century. An ageing population is a natural aspiration for any society, but it is not enough on its own (BRASIL, 2007).

Living longer is important as long as we can add quality to the additional years of life. This raises the following challenges for Public Health, as recognized by the World Health Organization.

(a)   how to maintain independence and an active life as we age?

(b)   how to strengthen health prevention and promotion policies, especially those aimed at the elderly?

(c)   How can we maintain and/or improve our quality of life as we age?

We need to find ways of incorporating the elderly into our society, change concepts that have already taken root and use new technologies, with innovation and wisdom, in order to achieve fairness and democracy in the distribution of services and facilities for the fastest-growing population group in our country, the elderly (BRASIL, 2007).

Concern about the elderly population is a matter of public health, which is a reflection of the increased interest in research in the area of public health and ageing in Brazil. Currently, a large number of studies cover topics such as health policies for the elderly and the use of medication, dependency and family care, violence of all kinds against the elderly, an anthropological approach to ageing, social inequalities and the health of the elderly, as well as population-based studies conducted in different communities and in the country as a whole.

Every year another 650,000 elderly people are added to the Brazilian population. We have wasted a lot of time believing that we were still a young country, without giving due credit to the demographic information that showed and projected the ageing of our population. With this study we intend to contribute to the expansion and consolidation of debates on these challenges (BRASIL, 2007).

3.10 Positive Effects of Physical and Mental Activity in the Treatment of Depression in the Elderly

Not a few studies have shown that physical and mental activity can be used to delay and even attenuate the process of decline in organic functions that is observed with ageing in longevity.

In addition, physical and mental activity leads to quality ageing, as it promotes improvements in respiratory capacity, cardiac reserve, reaction time, muscle strength, recent memory, cognition and social skills (CARDOSO JR, 1996).

According to the same author, physical and mental activity should be carried out preventively, i.e. before the disease shows its clinical manifestations. Rehabilitative interventions should be programmed to meet the needs of each individual and, in this way, physical activity should be maintained regularly throughout life so that the individual can enjoy improvements in quality of life and increased longevity. In addition, physical and mental activity leads the individual to greater social participation, resulting in a good level of biopsychophysical well-being, factors which contribute to improving their quality of life.

During physical and mental activity, bendorphine and dopamine are released by the body, providing a tranquilizing and analgesic effect on the regular practitioner, who often benefits from a relaxing after-effort effect and, in general, manages to maintain a more stable state of psychosocial equilibrium in the face of threats from the external environment (CARDOSO JR, 1996).

However, it is worth highlighting the importance of discerning between the concept of physical activity, which is a generic expression that can be defined as any bodily movement, produced by the skeletal muscles, that results in energy expenditure greater than resting levels. While physical exercise (one of its main components) is a planned, structured and repetitive physical activity that has the ultimate or intermediate goal of increasing or maintaining health/physical fitness.

Mental activity is an internal reconstruction of external operations with things and people, mediated by instruments and signs, mainly those of language, where the capacity for reflection and judgment, and therefore development, is born (CARDOSO JR, 1996).

According to the above, we can see that psychological changes are extrinsically linked to quality of life and play a major role in old age, requiring special attention (CARDOSO JR., 1996).

To talk about the elderly is to talk about our roots, and to talk about man in his essence, and human issues, and everything that emerges from being a person and their capacity for listening, respect, humility, empathy and, above all, human growth. The study was not intended to seek solutions for the world, but to reflect on this reality, which is present in the daily lives of families and communities.

4 METHODOLOGICAL PATH

Below, I outline the way in which this approach to reality is achieved in practice. The research is the result of a qualitative study which, in addition to identifying the incidence and prevalence of depression among the elderly, will also seek to answer specific questions which cannot be quantified. The research is qualitative because it works with meanings, beliefs, values, in a deeper space of human relationships (MINAYO, 1994).

Below I present the paths taken to achieve the objectives of the work.

4.1 Type of research

This is an exploratory, interpretative study of a qualitative nature, using the technique of Content Analysis to process the data.

In qualitative research, Content Analysis (CA), as a method for organizing and analyzing data, has some characteristics. Firstly, it is accepted that its focus is on qualifying the subject's experiences, as well as their perceptions of a given object and its phenomena (BARDIN, 2006).

Field research involves observing facts and phenomena exactly as they occur in reality, collecting data about them and, finally, analyzing and interpreting this data, based on a consistent theoretical foundation, with the aim of understanding and explaining the problem being researched (SEVERINO, 2002).

We opted for a qualitative approach to answer particular questions that cannot be quantified. This choice is justified because we wanted to work with the meanings that people attribute to their experiences in the social world, as well as the meanings attributed to them by the segment of interest (MINAYO, 1994).

The proposal is to promote a reflection on depression in the elderly, with the aim of identifying the functional impact of depression on them, proposing physical and mental activity as an aid to its treatment.

4.2 Research location

The study was carried out in a Basic Health Unit - UBS, located in the southern region of the city of Sao Paulo. This location was chosen by the Southern Regional Health Coordination - CRSSUL, due to the large number of elderly people who make up the community in its area of coverage.

According to information from the Primary Care Information System (SIAB), the UBS selected for this study covers an area of 21,968 registered people, of whom 7.99% are elderly, 3.31% male and 4.68% female.

In order to serve the registered population, the UBS has 6 health teams, which covers 6 geographical areas. Each area is made up of 4 micro-areas, totaling 24 micro-areas.

The sample consisted of 50 elderly people aged 60 or over, regardless of whether or not they had ever suffered from depression.

Participants were selected randomly, making up a total of 50 elderly people, from the elderly registered at the UBS mentioned above and who met the following inclusion criteria.

- You must be aged 60 or over;

- Whether or not they have ever been depressed;

- Have the cognitive ability to answer the questions posed by the researcher;

- Agree to take part in the study.

We emphasize that for the sample we had elderly people representing the 6 coverage areas of the UBS.

4.3 Data Collection Procedures

The elderly were approached by means of a questionnaire, in compliance with the precepts of CNS Resolution 466/2012, and only after the favorable opinions of the Research Ethics Committee of IAMSPE and the Municipal Government of the State of São Paulo (Annex I).

The questionnaire was administered in the homes of the elderly participants during home visits, where the researcher was accompanied at all times by a member of the health team responsible for the area and micro-area covered.

At this point, the researcher was introduced to the elderly person, who formalized the invitation to take part in the study.

After agreeing, the elderly person signed the Informed Consent Form (Appendix A).

The visits took place in such a way as to involve all the areas belonging to the UBS's catchment area.

In addition to signing the Informed Consent Form (Appendix A), the interviewees answered a few questions according to a previously established script (Appendix B).

4.4 Instruments and Data Collection

Considering the object of study and the proposed objectives, the most appropriate technique for data collection was the application of three questionnaires made up of three parts, described below:

The first part presented data on the participant's identity, such as age, date of birth, state of birth, address, length of time living, telephone number, marital status, gender, whether they were retired, and their previous and current occupation (Appendix B).

The second part contains information on socio-economic, cultural and family composition data (Appendix C).

The third and final part of the first questionnaire was made up of 18 objective questions related to everyday feelings, giving the degree of importance to each of these feelings, followed by an open question in which we asked the elderly person what depression was for them (Appendix D).

The average recording time between the question and the answer to the open-ended question was approximately 10 minutes. The variation in time depended on the participant's answer; when they were objective in their response, the time did not exceed five minutes.

For this open-ended question, permission was requested to record it on audio, which was then transcribed in full and the originality of the participants' speeches was maintained.

Finally, we administered what we also call the second questionnaire: the Abbreviated *Geriatric Depression Scale* (GDS) - 15-question version (Appendix II).

These scales are useful quick assessment tools to facilitate the identification of depression in the elderly. They are used to measure the degree of impairment in each case.

Some of the instruments used were filled in by the research participants themselves, while others were filled in by a family member, carer or guardian who was present at the time of the visit and the questionnaires were administered. In some cases, even the researcher himself, as indicated below:

- The instruments filled in by the research participants accounted for 75%, while the instruments filled in by the participants' relatives and companions accounted for 20%, and the other instruments filled in by the researcher accounted for 5%.

Data was collected from April 1st to June 30th, 2014.

4.5 Data Analysis and Discussion

According to Flik (2009) and Minayo (2006), qualitative research requires the researcher to be technically prepared and impartial in their reading, in order to understand what the other person values and not what the researcher would like to find, as well as making it possible to tabulate the existing quantitative variables, a fact that occurred in this study in the axes: gender correlating the number of women and men with depression, age, number of patients with the pathology and number of elderly people with the pathology who perform physical exercises.

Based on the research objectives, the theoretical framework used to analyze the data collected was Content Analysis.

According to Bardin (2009), Content Analysis involves three chronological stages: [...] "Pre-Analysis; Exploration of the Material; Treatment of the Results".

In the Pre-Analysis phase, as recommended by the author, a general "floating" reading was carried out, where the first general contact with the data to be analyzed was established, systematizing the initial ideas.

The material was then explored, a phase which required a long period of dedication on the part of the researcher, during which the data was coded. From the reading, passages were highlighted in order to grasp the meanings and senses expressed by the words described by the participants.

The categories and subcategories were grouped by themes and items of meaning, which allowed the first categories to emerge from the content of the answers, aggregating and qualifying their meanings, facilitating their interpretation in search of impressions, representations, emotions, knowledge and expectations.

Categorization refers to the classification of groups of recording units with generic titles and common elements, for later inference. Inference is the purpose of content analysis (deducing through reasoning) (BARDIN, 2009).

When the results were processed, they were grouped into three categories: Meaning of depression; Feelings of depression and Symptoms of depression.

These categories emerged from the analysis of the content that emerged from the participants' responses, seeking out symbolic impressions and representations, as well as emotions, knowledge and expectations (MINAYO, 2006).

The answers to the questionnaires were identified using Arabic numerals, which run from 01 to 50 sequentially, plus the letter "I" representing the word "elderly" placed before the numeral.

4.6 Characterization of the Research Participants

The systematization of the data from the first questionnaire (parts I and II) shows the following results in relation to the socio-demographic profile of the 50 elderly participants in the survey.

> **Gender**

Of the 50 participants, 29 were female and 21 male.

> **Marital status**

As for marital status, 2% of these elderly people are single, 22% widowed, 25% married and 1% divorced.

> **Age**

Social aging is related to the norms that control the performance of certain activities or tasks of the age group, based on an age criterion, and which give meaning to each person's life. It can be seen that the age of the participants was between 60-90 years, of which 44% were between 60-70 years, 38% between 71-80 years and 18% between 81-90 years.

> **Living time:**

On average, 23.4% of the participants have lived in the same place for more than 50 years.

> **Type of home**

50% of the participants live in their own home, 30% live with relatives and 20% pay rent.

> **Family Income**

It is clear from the data collected at this stage that the dependence of the elderly is one of the factors that trigger depression. 36% of the participants have a monthly income of one minimum wage, 13% have no income and 51% concealed the information.

> **Health Plan**

Among the participants in the survey, 10.5% had private health insurance or were dependent on a family member's health insurance. While 89.5% do not have a private health plan.

> **Education**

42.9% have completed primary school (represented by the first 4 years of primary school); 24.3% started primary school but didn't finish; 22.1% never went to school but were literate; 10.7% are not literate.

> **State of birth**

Of the 50 participants in the survey, 5 were born in Sao Paulo; 44 were born in other Brazilian states; 1 was born in Buenos Aires/Argentina.

> **Who you live with**

100% of the participants live with family members.

> **Loss of children**

It was observed that the loss of loved ones such as children, wives and husbands indicates one of the imminent conditions for depression in the elderly. We found that 10% of these elderly people had lost one child, 7% had lost two children and 2% of those interviewed had lost three children. While 30% had lost husbands and wives.

This data was not intended to explore all the factors that contribute to depression in ageing. However, the data obtained shows that these factors can influence not only depression, but also keep the elderly away from possibilities that could prevent situations such as depression.

5 RESULTS AND DISCUSSION

The systematization of the data collected refers to the third and final part of the first questionnaire (part III), which refers to 18 objective questions related to the real feelings of the elderly. This part of the questionnaire was designed with the aim of detecting any signs of low self-esteem, which would indicate the possibility of a depressive state. In this way, all the alternatives were made up of negative phrases. The participant had the following options to choose from: **Never; A little; All the time.** The following results were obtained from this part of the questionnaire:

> Never 52%; A little 45%; 3% All the time;

With regard to the participants who were part of the 3% who marked **all** the **time,** we observed that they were already being followed up by the health team in their area, others in the reference specialty outpatient clinic. Only 1 participant appeared as a newcomer. For this last case, a visit from the area's health team was immediately requested so that the follow-up process could begin.

For the Abbreviated Geriatric *Depression Scale* (Gds) 15-question version, which we call the second questionnaire. In this instrument, the results expressed by the participant reflect their feelings during the last week prior to the application of the scale. As already mentioned, this scale aims to verify the presence of depression, as well as the degree to which it is present. A score of 0 to 5 is considered normal, 6 to 10 indicates mild depression and 11 to 15 classifies depression as severe. After analyzing the results, the following findings were obtained: 97% of the participants' scores classified them as normal; 3% had mild depression.

The following are the categories and subcategories that emerged during the full transcription of the speeches of the elderly participants in the research.

The results of this study were grouped into three categories. The first category "Meaning of depression" is divided into the subcategories "translation of the inexplicable" and "relationship with illness". The second category "Feeling of depression" is described in two subcategories "suffering" and "imaginary" and the third category is translated as "Symptoms of depression" represented by the categories "sadness" and "relationship with loss".

The Subcategories are translated from the regrouping and final configuration of the categories, which are translated through the researcher's perception of the research participant's feelings.

1.1 Category I - Meaning of depression

This category shows the meaning of depression for the research participants, acquired through the experience of each research subject during the process of coping with the illness. This aspect allows us to know the essence and value that the person translates as a way of expressing their meaning.

The subcategory "translation of the inexplicable" shows in the interviewees' speeches the lack of clarity about depression, which they understood as something that is still unclear, but with some damage to the human being to be unraveled, as shown in chart 2.

1.2 Depression from the perspective of the elderly.

Table 2: Category I - Meaning of depression

1ª Subcategory	Interviewee's words
Translating the inexplicable	(I - 1) "It's the end of everything"
	(I - 15) "I don't know, but I live with my sister who is very upbeat, in a good mood, I don't think anyone would get sick with her".
	(I - 16) "I don't know what it is, but I'm sure I'll never suffer from it again. Life is all good to me!"
	(I - 20) "I don't know, but I've seen some very strange people who said they had depression. They were very distant from everything and very sad."
	(I - 24) "I don't know"
	(I - 30) "I don't know. I have no idea".
	(I - 34) "I've never had it. I don't know what it is".
	(I - 41) (43)" I don't know. I imagine it's not a good thing.
	(I - 41) (43) "I don't know what no is".
	(I - 45)" I don't know. If that's what my wife had, it was very annoying".

Source: Questionnaire answered by the elderly participants in the survey.

The second subcategory reveals that the majority of the participants in the survey understand depression as a physiological response, categorized by the **subcategory of Disease**, where they also report it as being little known, a woman's disease, which makes people sadder and most of which makes them want to die, as shown in Chart 3.

Chart 3: Category I - Meaning of depression

2ª Subcategory	Interviewee's words
	(I - 7)"I think depression is a little-known illness, we don't know when we're suffering from it, but I was a little sad for a few months and I got better when I started taking the medication and going for walks with the group here at the Unit".
	(I - 8)"That's a woman's thing to me, a macho man doesn't have that."
	(I - 10) "I think everyone in my family has had a bit of this illness, we've had a problematic family in everything. I think depression is because of the problems we can't solve."
	(I - 17)"I know it's something that makes people feel very bad and sad".
	(I - 18)" I think it's a disease that depresses people".
Disease relationship	(I - 21)"I know it's a disease that makes people who have it very withdrawn, but I don't have that with my old man!"
	(I - 25)"For me, depression is the stuff of people who have nothing to do"
	(I - 29)"I've been told that it's when you want to be very lonely, or you want to die. I don't know, I've never had it.
	(I - 33)"I know it's a disease that kills very quickly and worse, they say it passes from father to son".
	(I - 35)" I know because I've had friends who've had it. It's a very sad illness that leaves you very lonely. That's why I don't stop, I always try to do one thing or another, play dominoes or be with friends".

Source: Questionnaire answered by the elderly participants in the survey.

We can understand that most of the interviewees understand depression as something that is not good, as a process that can lead to death, restlessness, suffering and emotional exhaustion.

Depression affects people at the interface of their daily lives, where it translates into signs and symptoms representing changes in a person's behavior, attitude, coping and even disorder. For

Silva, Andrade, Neri and Melo (2015), depression is one of the processes that involves health problems in the population today, affecting mainly the elderly population, as they are more vulnerable due to their life trajectory.

1.3 Category II - Feeling depressed

The feeling of depression category tells us how the study participants perceive or feel about depression in themselves or in others close to them, emphasizing the habits, manners and conduct they experience on a daily basis. The majority portray their feelings as suffering after some kind of trauma, situations in which they experienced losses or defeats, represented by the subcategory suffering, as shown in Chart 4.

Table 4 - Category II - Feeling depressed

3ª Subcategory	Interviewee's words
Suffering	(I - 02)"My son *has had it,* it was terrible. What helped was the medication and when he started doing capoeira".
	(I - 03)"I wouldn't wish it on my worst enemy".
	(I - 04)"It was something that happened, and it almost ended my life, my daughter, I'll tell you something, I don't think I ever had that, but sometimes I think my husband died of it".
	(I - 11)"I've never had it, I think because I don't stay still. I'm always doing something different, moving around, but I know it's really bad, really sad, you know?
	(I - 12)"I think every widower is depressed. It's very sad to be alone".
	(I -14)"Just thinking that I've grown old, I've suffered a lot, you know? Worse still, without learning anything about life, that makes me sad, that's depression"?
	(I - 38)"I know why my wife had it. I thought she would die of sadness. After taking a lot of medication and starting to walk, dance and do other activities with the women's group here at the health center, she improved a lot".

Source: Questionnaire answered by the elderly participants in the survey.

The lack of understanding of the symptoms, the causes, the damage and the way to care for depression reveals that the participants in the survey have an imaginary knowledge of the disorder, describing it as something that is acquired through the results of each person's life situation, within their history from the inside out, which grows from each person's daily confrontations, thus the subcategory reveals the Imaginary, as shown in Chart 5.

Table 5: Category II - Feeling depressed

4th Subcategory	Interviewee's words
	(I - 13 "It's a very bad thing".
The imaginary	(I - 9)"I had it when I became a widow, but I got better by taking some medication and taking part in activities such as walks, trips and hiking groups back home". (I - 27) "I think I've had it, but I managed to get over it. I felt very depressed after the death of my son and it got worse after I became a widower. I thought I would have died too if it hadn't been for my children. They encouraged me to take part in the activities here at the health center. Today I don't stop taking part in all the activities. (I - 28)"I don't like being so dependent on family members. I'd like to be more independent, but my situation forces me to be subject to things like my financial situation, my old age and my limitations. I can't even walk properly anymore". (I - 32)"I had depression when I was widowed, but my four children did everything they could to help me get better. I believe that nobody gets well if they don't want to. There's no family, no medicine or doctor that can help. Today I'm well and I'm always moving with the walking group and other groups here at the health center and with my neighbors". (I- 37)"I've had it when my two children died, but my husband and my family have been very good to me. I don't know if I'm cured, but I don't feel like dying anymore. I think the medicines and exercises I do here at the UBS have helped me a lot". (I- 40)"I've never had it, but I know exactly what it is. I helped look after someone with depression, she was very down, she just wanted to kill herself". (I- 42)"When I arrived here in Sao Paulo, I went through a lot of difficulties, the doctor gave me some medication and said I had this thing. I took the

<table>
<tr><td></td><td>medication, but I think it was the love and patience of my children that cured me".

(I - 44)"When I left my country I went through several painful processes, I even thought that my life had been left behind, I didn't master the language, I didn't know anyone here in Brazil. I think I had this kind of depression. I didn't take any medication, but it was complicated. I think my husband's attention and understanding helped me get out of this situation".

(I - 46)"I've never had these things, but there are several people in my family who have. I think there's a lot of this in Minas Gerais. And the people there aren't lazy, they just love to dance".</td></tr>
</table>

Source: Questionnaire answered by the elderly participants in the survey.

Through the words of the interviewees, we can see that they understand depression to be some kind of disorder that affects the individual, disorganizing their physiological state, where changes in behavior, attitude, fear, euphoria, isolation and pain are the signs and symptoms presented by them, as a way of changing the person's natural state, sometimes requiring the intervention of medication.

These data could encourage the reduction of helplessness to a direct effect of organic variables (MAIER and GRAU, 1982).

In this sense, the symptoms of depression (physiological or otherwise) can be the direct result of a malfunction in the body (ABREU, 2014).

Emphasizing that depression has become an aggravating factor for mental health today, leading to people withdrawing from activities they have previously performed, compromising their social and collective lives (WHO, 2009).

This social breakdown often leads to personal isolation, which implies future pathology, diagnosed as depression, affecting thousands of people who experience this situation (WHO, 2009).

Despite these findings, we can identify in the interviewees' speeches, the difficulty of the person who is suffering and going through this phase, their own perception in correlating personal changes that indicate the disease, where they are not aware of the alternatives to be able to promote actions for their self-care (WHO, 2009).

1.4 Category III - Depressive symptoms

This category highlighted signs and symptoms such as crying, sadness, pain and sleepiness. Clearly demonstrated in the interviewees' speeches, these are situations that shake the emotional state, where some seek medical help to resolve the symptoms and others are urged by family members to help themselves. This category will be dealt with under the subcategory behavioral changes, as shown in Chart 6.

Table 6: Category III - Symptoms of depression

Subcategory	Interviewee's words
Behavior change	(I - 06)"So one of my daughters had some of these symptoms for a long time, I took her to several doctors and they just gave her lots of medication that made her sleep and eat a lot. She was almost twice her weight and when she died she was so sad it was painful. I too sometimes feel endless sadness, but it gets better when I do activities that force me to move my skeleton. I think it's a disease that kills.
	(I - 09)"My doctor referred me to a psychologist because I was a bit weepy and sometimes very nervous. I think depression is a very sad thing.
	(I - 36)"Doctor, I think I was born with it. After I became a widow I went off the deep end. I feel so lonely, even when I'm with other people. Sometimes I'm very sleepy and I sleep for days, and then I feel even worse when I don't want to sleep. And so I go on with my life.
	(I - 50)"I feel tired, sleepy, sometimes agitated, I don't understand what's happening..."

Source: Questionnaire answered by the elderly participants in the survey.

In the speeches, we can analyze various aspects when presenting the signs and symptoms of rapid onset. Most of the time it is ignored, initially by the patient themselves, by family members and even by the health professional who initially sees the patient.

According to Oliveira (2006), elderly people with symptoms of depression are often neglected when it comes to diagnosing and treating depression, which alters their quality of life, as well as increasing the economic burden on health services, due to its direct and indirect costs.

Despite its clinical relevance, depressive symptomatology in the elderly is little verified and valued by health professionals (SOUZA, 2007).

From this perspective, nursing can play a fundamental role in offering care based on a clinical and reflective approach to the elderly and their care, in order to preserve their physical and mental health and their moral, intellectual and spiritual development, in conditions of autonomy and dignity.

Today's health facilities, in line with public health policies, have a lot to offer and contribute to enabling the elderly population to get through this time of their lives with a little more quality, which would consequently improve their self-esteem and prevent many health problems such as depression.

The UBS where the research was carried out has planned health actions specifically for its community, taking into account socio-economic situations and prioritizing risk groups.

Concerned with the population as a whole, and specifically with the elderly population, the UBS currently maintains a special program where the elderly, in addition to the traditional care provided by the health team, can also count on daily integrative health practices, such as walking, Liang Gong, Tai Chi Chuan, circular dance, gardening and games that help activate memory.

5   FINAL CONSIDERATIONS

This research has enabled us to point out some of the contributions that physical and mental activities make to the lives of the elderly who practice them, thus demonstrating the importance of these activities as a strategy for strengthening the patient and the family, as well as rescuing the self-esteem of the elderly.

With the aim of identifying the functional impact of depression in elderly people attending a specific Basic Health Unit, we sought to identify social factors as having a strong impact on triggering depression. We realized that the process of depression in the elderly is evident and growing, requiring strategies that promote changes in attitude and behavior.

To this end, it is necessary to build ways to stimulate and challenge the elderly to work with possibilities that make it more difficult for them to be vulnerable to the development of depression.

The conditions of income, housing, age, among others, and especially adequate support in coping with loss, were shown to be factors that indirectly and directly interfere with dignified ageing.

From this perspective, it is important for family members to provide emotional and psychological support, encouraging the elderly to join in and practice activities that occupy their time and help prevent the loss or impairment of their physical and motor mobility, minimizing emotional suffering, and contributing to the recovery of family and social ties, strengthening solidarity support networks, according to the Ministry of Health in the Pact for Health - Pact in Defense of Life. Thus favoring aging with greater quality.

This emphasizes that physical and mental activity is essential both in prevention and after the onset of depression, as it has a positive influence on coping with a depressive process.

The reports showed that the start of physical and mental activity, as well as social interaction, stimulated the body, directly influencing the prevention of depression.

In the course of the research, it was found through the speech, as well as the reports of family members, that the majority of elderly people who had a depressive episode, obtained a significant improvement from the beginning of physical and mental activity, that is, bodily activity leads directly to mental exercise, which contributes as an aid in the treatment of depression in the elderly.

It has also been shown that elderly people who do physical and mental activities report that there are significant influences on the prevention of depression.

The conclusion of this study corroborates the statements made by some of the authors cited above, when they state that physical and mental activity not only significantly improves the physiological process of ageing, but can also be carried out in a preventative manner, as well as in the face of an already installed depressive state, or in order to help with treatment, and should be maintained within the possibilities of the elderly person on a regular basis, favoring and stimulating social interaction and participation, thus resulting in biopsychophysical and social well-being, improving quality of life.

At the end of this study, it was possible to understand that one of the factors contributing to depression in the elderly, among the factors already listed, is the decrease in physical and mental activity, because with the arrival of old age the individual feels a loss of prestige due to the loss of productivity in society, isolating themselves from the people they live with and plunging into a process of loneliness, abandoning daily activities which directly interfere with physical and motor mobility.

This study draws attention not only to the need for professionals in multidisciplinary teams to acquire technical and scientific knowledge about mental health, but also to the need for family members to seek guidance on the issue of the illness, especially about the prejudice that depression produces: the vast majority of elderly people easily confuse depression with old age, and do not believe that the elderly person really has an illness, but is simply in the process of normal ageing, a term scientifically called "senescence".

6   REFERENCES

ALMEIDA, O. P.; LOFER, B.; FILHO, E.C.M. Depression in the elderly: a review. **Rev. Paul. Méd**, 1990. 108p.

ALVES, [B. J. G.] et al. Health-related physical fitness in the elderly: influence of water aerobics. **Revista Brasileira de Medicina do Esporte**, v. 10, n. 1, p. 31-37, 2004.

ANGELOTTI, G. Cognitive-behavioral treatment of depression. In:CAMON, A. A. (Org.). *Depression and Psychosomatics*. Sao Paulo: Pioneira Thomson Learning, 2011. 177 p.

ANTUNES, [H. K.] M.*et al.* Cognitive Alterations in Elderly as a Result of Systematized Physical Exercise. **Revista da Sobama**.6(1): 27-33, 2001.

ANTUNES, [H. K.] M, *et al.* The effect of an aerobic physical conditioning program for normal elderly people on performance in neuropsychological tests. In: *XVI Reunião anual da FESBE* : Caxambu - MG, 2001. 272 p.

BALLONE, G.J. **Depression in the Elderly**. In. PsiqWeb General Psychiatry. Available at <http://www.psiqweb.med.br/geriat/depidoso.html>. Accessed on December 20, 2015.

BARDIN, L. **Content Analysis.** Lisbon, Portugal: Ediçoes 70, 2006.

BERQUÓ, E. **Algumas considerações demogràficas sobre o envelhecimento da populaçao no Brasil** - paper presented at the International Congress on Population Ageing - an agenda for the end of the century, mimeo, Brasilia, 2006.

BRAZIL. Ministry of Health. **Ageing and health of the elderly**. Secretariat of Health Care, Department of Primary Care. - Brasilia: Ministry of Health, 2007.

BRAZIL. Ministry of Health. **Statute of the Elderly**. 2ª ed. Rev. - Brasilia: Editora **do** Ministério da Saùde, 2007. 70 p.

CALDAS, [G. A.] & cols. Depression in the elderly. **Revista Informaçao Psiquiàtrica**. 3(1): 2329, 1994.

COMER, [R. J.] **Psychology of Special Behavior**. 4th ed. Rio de Janeiro: LTC, 2003.

CAMON, V. A. A. Depression as a vital process. In:CAMON V. A. A. (Org.). *Depression and Psychosomatics* (p. 1-44). Sao Paulo: Pioneira Thomson Learning, 2001. 44 p.

CARDOSO, J.R. **Physical activities for the elderly**. A terceira idade. 5(4): 9-21, 1992.

CORRÊA, A.C.O. Depression and suicide in the elderly: a crucial issue in psychogeriatrics. **J Bras Psiquiatr**. 45:149-157, 1996.

CARVALHO, V. F. C.; FERNANDEZ, M.E.D. Depression in the elderly. In: PAPALÉ-ONETTO, M. (ed.) **Gerontologia**. Sao Paulo; Rio de Janeiro: Atheneu, 1996.

DAS GUPTA, K. M. D. Treatment of depression in elderly patients. **JAMA Brazil**. 5(1): 69-76, 2001.

FLICK U. **Introduction to qualitative research**.3ª ed. Porto Alegre: Artmed, 2009.

FREITAS, E. V. et al. Tratado **de Geriatria e Gerontologia**. Rio de Janeiro: Guanabara Koogan, 2006.

GEIS, P. P. **Physical activity and health in old age: theory and practice**. 5th ed. Porto Alegre: Artmed, 2003.

GORESTEIN, C. et al. **Clinical assessment scales in psychiatry and psychopharmacology**. Sao Paulo: Lemos Editorial, 2000. 438 p.

KAPLAN, H. I.; SODOCK, B. J.; GREBB, J.A. **Compendium of Psychiatry - behavioral science and clinical psychiatry**. 7th ed. Porto Alegre: Artmed, 2003.

LAFER, B. & Amaral, J. A. M. S. **Depression in the life cycle**. Porto Alegre: Artes Médicas, 2000.

MARIN-NETO, J.A. et al. Physical activities: scientifically proven "medicine"? **The Third Age**. 10(6): 34-43, 1995.

MARQUEZ FILHO, E. Physical activity in the aging process. **The Third Age**. 10(6): 62-69, 1995.

MATSUDO, S. M. Physical activity in the promotion of health and quality of life in aging. **Revista Brasileira de Educaçao Fisica e Esporte**, v. 20, n. 1, p. 135-137, 2006.

MINAYO,M. C. S. **O desafio do conhecimento: pesquisa qualitativa em saùde**. Sao Paulo: Hucitec; 2006.

NASCIMENTO, I. Unipolar depression: a review. Rio de Janeiro. **Revista Informaçao Psiquiâtrica**. 18(3): 75-83, 1999.

NERI, A L. Psychological Theories of Aging. In: FREITAS, E V. et al. **Tratado de Geriatria e Gerontologia**. Rio de Janeiro: Guanabara Koogan, 2002.

OLIVEIRA,D.A.A.P.; GOMES, L.; OLIVEIRA, R.F. Prevalência de depressao em idosos que freqüam centros de convivência. **Rev Saùde Pùblica**.40(4): 734-6, 2006.

WORLD HEALTH ORGANIZATION (OMS). **The role of physical activity in healthy ageing**. Florianópolis, 2006.

PORCU, Mauro et al. Comparative study on the prevalence of depressive symptoms in the elderly.

ActaScientiarum. V. 24, 2002. Available at:

<http://periodicos.uem.br/ojs/index.php/ActaSciHealthSci/article/view/2498>. Accessed on: November 25, 2015.

PY, L.; TREIN, F. Finitude and Infinitude: dimensions of time in the experience of aging. In: FREITAS, E.V. et al. **Tratado de Geriatria**. Rio de Janeiro: Guanabara Koogan, 2002. 1021 p.

NATIONAL SURVEY BY SAMPLE OF HOUSEHOLDS - Summary of Indicators, 2012. Available at:

<http://www.ibge.gov.br/home/estatistica/populacao/trabalhoerendimento/pnad2013 accessed on 05/03/2015>. Accessed on: October 10, 2015.

RIBEIRO, M. A.M. et al. Prevalence of depression in full-time institutionalized elderly. **Rer. Psiquiatr. Clin.** Sao Paulo, 1994.

SÂO PAULO. State Health Secretariat. **Manual de Assistência de Enfermagem a Saùde da Pessoa Idosa** - SMS/SP - 4ª ed. Sao Paulo, 2012.

SÂO PAULO. Secretaria da Saù, Coordenaçao da Atença Bàsica. **Manual de Atençâo à Pessoa Idosa. Secretaria da Saù, Coordenaçao da Atençâo Bàsica/ Estratégia Saù da Familia**. - 2 ed - Sao Paulo: SMS, 2012. 66 p.

SEVERINO, A. J. **Metodologia do trabalho cientifico**. Sao Paulo: Cortez, 2002.

SIQUEIRA, M. E. C. **Teorias Sociológicas do Envelhecimento**.Tratado de Geriatria e Gerontologia. Rio de Janeiro: Guanabara Koogan, 2002.

SILVA, E. M. M. et al. Diseases of the Elderly Patient. **PesqBrasOdontopedClinIntegr**. v. 7, n. 1, p. 83-88, 2007.

SOUSA R. L, et al. Validity and reliability of the Geriatric Depression Scale in the identification of depressed elderly in a general hospital. **J Bras Psiquiatr**. 56(2): 102-7, 2007.

STOPPE-JR, A. Clinical characteristics of depression in the elderly. In: FORLENZA,O.V. and ALMEIDA, O. P. Sao Paulo: Lemos Editorial, 1997.

TAVARES, L. A. T. A **depressao como "mal-estar" contemporàneo: medicalização e existência do sujeito depressivo**. Sao Paulo: Editora UNESP; Sao Paulo: Cultura Acadêmica, 2010.

WAGNER,G. A. Treatment of depression in the elderly beyond fluoxetine hydrochloride **Rev. Saùde Pùblica**. 49:20, 2015.

SANTAREM, J. M. Bases Fisiológicas do Exercicio, na saù, na doença, e no envelhecimento, 2002,

Available at: http://www.saudetotal.com>. Accessed on: October 10, 2015.

7 APPENDICES

Appendix A - Informed Consent Form

TCLE - FREE AND INFORMED CONSENT FORM

Title: "The Importance of Physical and Mental Activity in Helping to Treat Depression in the Elderly".

INVITATION

You are being invited as a volunteer to participate in the research: **The Importance of Physical and Mental Activity in Helping to Treat Depression in the Elderly**

We know the benefits of physical and mental activity as a way of improving quality of life, including for older people with certain age-specific illnesses, including depression.

This research aims to learn more about how depression occurs in the elderly, as well as how physical and mental activity can help to improve it, thus helping to treat depression.

To take part in the research, we will meet during a home visit by the researcher accompanied by the health team responsible for the area and micro-area of the health service - Unidade Bàsica de Saù. At this point you will be invited. If you accept, you will be interviewed. In order to get to know a little about your life story, we will try to find out the following information:

Name. Sex. Address. Age. Date of birth. State of birth. How long you have lived at this address. Telephone number. If married, single, widowed, divorced or other. Do you work, what do you do at the moment, if retired, what did you do before you retired. Do you have health insurance? If you studied, how far you managed to study. Do you live in your own home, rented, other. Do you have children, number of children, number of living children. Who do you live with, husband/partner, relatives or alone or other. If you don't live with family, how often do you visit them?

We will also ask you a few questions to find out how you feel about what life has been like emotionally, and we will apply two depression scales - the Beck Scale and the Geriatric Depression Scale, which are used to measure the severity of depressive cases.

We would like to inform you that the research will not pose any risk to you. During the research, if you present any need for follow-up, you will be referred and followed up for appropriate treatment by scheduling appointments following the flow of care of the unit and health team.

You are free to refuse to take part, and if any situation of embarrassment is identified, you can withdraw your consent or stop taking part at any time during the research. Your participation is voluntary and refusal to participate, or discontinuation of participation, will not result in any penalty or loss of the right to referral, follow-up and treatment.

All information collected about you is confidential and will remain confidential until the end of the research. Your name or material indicating your participation will not be

Unauthorized without your permission. You will not be identified in any publication that may result from this study. A copy of this informed consent form will be stored in the postgraduate department of IAMSPE - Instituto de Assistência Médica ao Servidor Pùblico estadual, where the researcher is a regularly enrolled student, and another copy will be given to you.

Your participation in the study will be at no cost to you and no additional financial compensation will be available.

You will be informed about the research in any way you wish. If you have any questions about the research, they can be clarified by the research nurse - Maria Socorro Cardoso dos Santos, ID card number 13.957.024-x, CPF 039.503.858-86. Resident at Condominio Marajoara sol, located at Avenida Interlagos, n° 492, bloco 3 Apartamento 133 Bairro, Jardim Marajoara - CEP 04660.000. The researcher can also be reached by telephone on (011) cell 9 89993085, or by sending messages to the following e-mail address: E-mail mariasocorro.cardoso@yahoo.com.br

If you have any questions about the ethics of the research, you can contact IAMSPE's Research Ethics Committee at: (11) 4573 - 8175, Rua Pedro de Toledo, n° 1.800, 14° andar - Vila Clementino, SP CEP-04039-901, where the researcher is duly enrolled in the Postgraduate Program. Interested parties may also contact the Research Ethics Committee of the SMS - Secretaria Municipal de Saù by telephone: 3397-2464 at Rua General Jardim, 36 1° andar, the place designated as the Co-Participating Institution of the Research Project, or by sending a message to the following e-mail address: E-mail:smscep@gmail.com.

I declare that I agree to take part in this study. I have received a copy of this informed consent form and have been given the opportunity to read it and clarify my doubts.

Name   Participant's signature Date

/Responsible

    NameMaria Socorro Cardoso dos / Date

Santos

Appendix B

Part I- Identification

IDENTIFICATION

Name:____

Age:

Date of Birth://

State of birth: _______________________________________

Address: ____

Living time: ____

Phone:____

Marital status:

(   ) Married

(   ) Married

(   ) Viùvo

(   ) Divorced

(   ) Separated

(   ) Single

Gender: (   ) Male (   ) Female

Retired: (   ) Yes (   ) No

Current Activity:Previous Activity

Appendix C

Part II - Sociodemographic, cultural and family composition data.

SOCIODEMOGRAPHIC, CULTURAL AND FAMILY COMPOSITION DATA

1. Do you have a health insurance plan? (   ) Yes () No, if yes, which one?

2. Education: (   ) Elementary School Complete ()   Elementary School Incomplete (   )

Complete High School (   )   Incomplete   High   School   ()   Complete
    Higher Education (   )

Incomplete Higher Education (   ) Postgraduate ( ) Master's Degree

( ) Doctorate (   ) Never attended school.

3. Dwelling: (   ) owned ()   rented ()   other Which?

4. Income: ( ) No Income ( ) 1 to 3 Minimum Wages (   ) 4 to 5 Minimum Wages

(   ) Above 6 minimum wages, how many?

5. Number of children: _______________

6. Number of living children:

7. Who do you live with?

(   ) with spouse

(   ) with family members

(   ) alone

(   ) others, With whom? _________________

8. Weekly family time: (   ) yes (   ) no, how often?

Appendix D

Part III - Feelings of the Elderly

DATA ON HOW THE ELDERLY REALLY FEEL

I think my life has been lived in vain.

1.   ( ) Never ()   A little (   ) All the time.

My future looks hopeless.

2.   ( ) Never ( ) A little ( ) All the time.

I feel like my life is meaningless.

3.   ( ) Never ( ) A little ( ) All the time.

I'm dissatisfied with my current life.

4.   ( ) Never ( ) A little ( ) All the time.

I have trouble making decisions.

5.   ( ) Never ( ) A little ( ) All the time.

I lost the pleasure I felt in life.

6.   ( ) Never ( ) A little ( ) All the time.

I feel sad, unmotivated and unhappy.

7.   ( ) Never ( ) A little ( ) All the time.

I feel isolated.

8.   ( ) Never ( ) A little ( ) All the time.

I feel tired.

9.   ( ) Never ( ) A little ( ) All the time.

It takes a lot of effort for me to do simple things.

10.   ( ) Never ()   A little (   ) All the time.

I don't want to shower.

11.   ( ) Never ()   A little (   ) All the time.

I feel like a failure.

12.   ( ) Never ()   A little () All the time.

I feel drained of energy, more dead than alive.

13.   ( ) Never ()   A little (   ) All the time.

My sleep is disturbed, I've been sleeping too little, insomnia, oversleeping or oversleeping.

14.   ( ) Never ()   A little (   ) All the time.

I waste time thinking about suicide.

15.   ( ) Never ()   A little (   ) All the time.

I don't want to talk to anyone.

16.   ( ) Never ()   A little (   ) All the time.

I feel depressed even when good things happen to me.

17.   ( ) Never ()   A little (   ) All the time.

Without trying to diet, I lost or gained weight.

18.   ( ) Never ()   A little (   ) All the time.

19.   What is depression for you?

8   Annexes

Annex I - *Abbreviated* **Geriatric Depression Scale (GDS)**

GERIATRIC

DEPRESSION SCALE **(GDS) (15-question version)**

It is a 15-question questionnaire with objective answers (yes or no) about how the elderly person has been feeling over the last week. The purpose of the Geriatric Depression Scale is to verify the presence of depression. It is not a substitute for a diagnostic interview carried out by mental health professionals. It is a useful quick assessment tool to facilitate the identification of depression in the elderly. Add 1 point to each affirmative answer. The questions cannot be changed, you must ask exactly what is on the instrument.

Evaluation of results: A score between 0 and 5 is considered normal, 6 to 10 indicates

mild depression and 11 to 15 severe depression.

Measures to be taken with the findings/results: high scores suggest referral for specific neuropsychological assessment.

ABBREVIATED GERIATRIC DEPRESSION SCALE

I.	Are you satisfied with your life?	Yes ( )	No ( )
2.	Have you interrupted many of your⅙ guests?	Yes ( )	No ()
J. Do you think your life is good?		Yes ( )	No ()
4.	Do you get bored often?	Yes ( )	No( )
	Do you feel good about life most of the time ?	Yes( )	No ( )
6.	Do you think something bad will happen to you?	Yes ( )	No ( )
7.Do you	feel cheerful most of the time?	Yes (jNo	( )
β. If you feel helpless Frequency?		Yes(⅙No	( )
9.	Would you rather stay at home than go out and do new things	? Yes{⅙No {	)
10.	Do you think you have more problems with your	memory than other people ? {	No ( )
11.	Do you think it's wonderful to be alive{a} ?	Yes ( )No{	)
Ii. Do you feel indifferent?		Yes ( )	No( )
12.	Do you feel full of energy?	Yes (JNo(	)
M. Do you feel hopeless?		Yes (JNo (	)
I S. Do you think others are luckier than you?		Yes ()	No()

Annex II - Opinion of the Research Ethics Committee - CEP IAMSPE and Prefeitura de Sao Paulo

INSTITUTO DE ASSISTÊNCIA
MÉDICA AO SERVIDOR
PÚBLICO ESTADUAL - IAMSPE
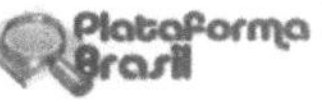

PARECER CONSUBSTANCIADO DO CEP

DADOS DO PROJETO DE PESQUISA

Título da Pesquisa: A Importância da Atividade Física e Mental no Auxílio ao Tratamento da Depressão em Idosos

Pesquisador: Maria Socorro Cardoso dos Santos

Área Temática:

Versão: 2

CAAE: 18933913.4.0000.5463

Instituição Proponente: Instituto de Assistência Médica ao Servidor Público Estadual - IAMSPE

Patrocinador Principal: Financiamento Próprio

DADOS DO PARECER

Número do Parecer: 490.989
Data da Relatoria: 10/12/2013

Apresentação do Projeto:
De acordo.

Objetivo da Pesquisa:
De acordo com o TCLE.

Avaliação dos Riscos e Benefícios:
Sem riscos.

Comentários e Considerações sobre a Pesquisa:
Sem considerações.

Considerações sobre os Termos de apresentação obrigatória:
De acordo.

Recomendações:

Conclusões ou Pendências e Lista de Inadequações:
Sem pendências.

Situação do Parecer:
Aprovado

Endereço: Rua Pedro de Toledo,1800 - 14° andar - Ala central - Sala 01
Bairro: Vila Clementino   **CEP:** 04.039-004
UF: SP   **Município:** SAO PAULO
Telefone: (11)4573-8175   **Fax:** (11)4573-8175   **E-mail:** cepiamspe@iamspe.sp.gov.br

INSTITUTO DE ASSISTÊNCIA
MÉDICA AO SERVIDOR
PÚBLICO ESTADUAL - IAMSPE

Necessita Apreciação da CONEP:

Não

Considerações Finais a critério do CEP:

O Colegiado acatou o parecer do relator.

SAO PAULO, 12 de Dezembro de 2013

Assinador por:
Gizelda Monteiro da Silva
(Coordenador)

Endereço: Rua Pedro de Toledo,1800 - 14° andar - Ala central - Sala 01
Bairro: Vila Clementino   CEP: 04.039-004
UF: SP   Município: SAO PAULO
Telefone: (11)4573-8175   Fax: (11)4573-8175   E-mail: cepiamspe@iamspe.sp.gov.br

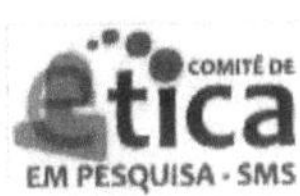

SECRETARIA MUNICIPAL DA SAÚDE DE SÃO PAULO - SMS/SP

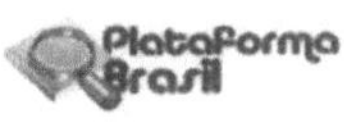

PARECER CONSUBSTANCIADO DO CEP

Elaborado pela Instituição Coparticipante

DADOS DO PROJETO DE PESQUISA

Título da Pesquisa: A Importância da Atividade Física e Mental no Auxílio ao Tratamento da Depressão em Idosos

Pesquisador: Maria Socorro Cardoso dos Santos

Área Temática:

Versão: 2

CAAE: 18933913.4.0000.5463

Instituição Proponente: Instituto de Assistência Médica ao Servidor Público Estadual - IAMSPE

Patrocinador Principal: Financiamento Próprio

DADOS DO PARECER

Número do Parecer: 509.165
Data da Relatoria: 06/02/2014

Apresentação do Projeto:

No Brasil e no mundo, o número de idosos tem aumentado, exigindo políticas públicas para o atendimento de suas necessidades específicas. A depressão é um estado clínico que acomete muitos idosos, exigindo um melhor entendimento para seu enfrentamento.

Trata-se de projeto de pesquisa que se propõe a analisar a relação entre o quadro de depressão e atividade mental e física nos idosos. Para tal, a autora pretende aplicar três questionários a 50 usuários da UBS da Vila das Belezas, situada região sul da cidade de São Paulo, com idade igual ou superior a 60 anos.

Diz tratar-se de um estudo interpretativo ancorado em pesquisa de campo. Os questionários serão aplicados durante visitas domiciliares que ocorrerão de forma a envolver todas as áreas e microareas pertencentes a área de abrangência desta UBS. Dois dos questionários contem questões sobre os aspectos socioeconômicos, culturais e de composição familiar e dois apresentam questões relacionadas diretamente com o quadro de depressão. Um deles é a Escala de Depressão de Beck.

Os questionários poderão ser preenchidos pelo sujeito de pesquisa, seu acompanhante ou pelo próprio pesquisador. Uma questão aberta será registrada em áudio com consentimento dos entrevistados, e as fitas transcritas na íntegra. Haverá um registro de observações.

Endereço: Rua General Jardim, 36 - 1° andar
Bairro: CENTRO   **CEP:** 01.223-010
UF: SP   **Município:** SAO PAULO
Telefone: (11)3397-2464   **E-mail:** smscep@gmail.com

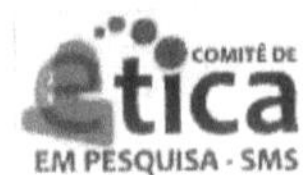

SECRETARIA MUNICIPAL DA SAÚDE DE SÃO PAULO - SMS/SP

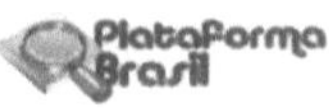

Continuação do Parecer: 509.165

Objetivo da Pesquisa:

OBJETIVO GERAL

Identificar o impacto funcional da depressão em idosos, buscando levantar subsídios, para estes demonstrar a importância da atividade física e mental como auxílio no tratamento da depressão em idosos.

OBJETIVOS ESPECÍFICOS

1. Caracterizar o perfil dos idosos frequentadores da UBS ¿ Unidade Básica de saúde;

2. Analisar o impacto das relações sociais e das atividades físicas em idosos;

3. Avaliar o impacto das relações sociais e das atividades físicas em idosos;

Avaliação dos Riscos e Benefícios:

A autora afirma não haver risco para os entrevistados, porém as perguntas contidas nos questionários podem suscitar situações constrangedoras, estressantes, de angústia e sofrimento para os sujeitos de pesquisa. Os sujeitos serão informados que poderão interromper a entrevista ou retirar seu consentimento caso sintam qualquer deconforto.

Comentários e Considerações sobre a Pesquisa:

A metodologia é adequada aos objetivos.

Considerações sobre os Termos de apresentação obrigatória:

A Folha de Rosto está corretamente preenchida, foram identificadas instituição proponente e coparticipante, autorização para realização da pesquisa foi adequadamente apresentada. Cronograma e orçamento detalhado estão adequados, os custos do projeto estarão a cargo do pesquisador. Há benefícios previstos na realização do estudo.

Termo de Consentimento Livre e Esclarecido (TCLE) foi considerado adequado após retificações.

Recomendações:

Enviar um adendo ao CEP da Instituição proponente a fim de que sejam informadas as alterações feitas ao projeto ora aprovado.

Conclusões ou Pendências e Lista de Inadequações:

Sem pendências ou inadequações.

Situação do Parecer:

Aprovado

Endereço: Rua General Jardim, 36 - 1º andar
Bairro: CENTRO   **CEP:** 01.223-010
UF: SP   **Município:** SAO PAULO
Telefone: (11)3397-2464   **E-mail:** smscep@gmail.com

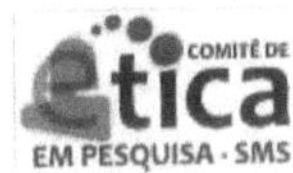

SECRETARIA MUNICIPAL DA SAÚDE DE SÃO PAULO - SMS/SP

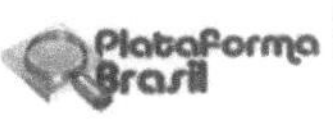

Necessita Apreciação da CONEP:

Não

Considerações Finais a critério do CEP:

Para início da coleta dos dados, o pesquisador deverá se apresentar na mesma instância que autorizou a realização do estudo (Coordenadoria, Supervisão, SMS/Gab, etc).

Se o projeto prever aplicação de TCLE, todas as páginas do documento deverão ser rubricadas pelo pesquisador e pelo voluntário e a última página assinada por ambos, conforme Carta Circular no 003/2011 da CONEP/CNS.

Salientamos que o pesquisador deve desenvolver a pesquisa conforme delineada no protocolo aprovado. Eventuais modificações ou emendas ao protocolo devem ser apresentadas ao CEP de forma clara e sucinta, identificando a parte do protocolo a ser modificada e suas justificativas. Lembramos que esta modificação necessitará de aprovação ética do CEP antes de ser implementada.

Ao pesquisador cabe manter em arquivo, sob sua guarda, por 5 anos, os dados da pesquisa, contendo fichas individuais e todos os demais documentos recomendados pelo CEP (Res. CNS 196/96 item IX. 2. e). De acordo com a Res. CNS 466/12, 0 pesquisador deve apresentar a este CEP/SMS os relatórios semestrais. O relatório final deverá ser enviado através da Plataforma Brasil, Ícone Notificação. Uma cópia digital (CD/DVD) do projeto finalizado deverá ser enviada à instância que autorizou a realização do estudo, via correio ou entregue pessoalmente, logo que o mesmo estiver concluído.

SAO PAULO, 06 de Março de 2014

____

Assinador por:
SIMONE MONGELLI DE FANTINI
(Coordenador)

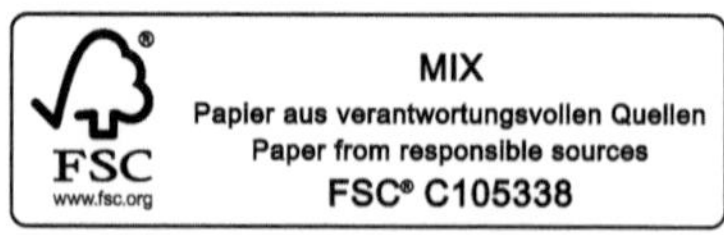

Printed by Books on Demand GmbH, Norderstedt / Germany